I0413014

Therapeutic Body And Skin Care Recipes

A DIY Guide For Homemade Baths
Products, Body Lotions, Whipped
Butters, Skin Creams, Herbal Salves,
Balms And Lot More,

SOPHIA FROST

ISBN-13:978-1511534529

ISBN-10:1511534524

DEDICATION

To Barry, thanks a million

TABLE OF CONTENT

INTRODUCTION 1

    Making Your Products Safe 3

    Natural Preservatives 5

BATH RECIPES 7

    Mud Bath 7

    Baking & Sea Salt Soda Detox Baths 8

    Apple Cider Vinegar (ACV) Detox Baths 9

    Skin Softening Milk Bath 10

    Baking Soda Detox Baths 11

    Muscle Relaxing Bath Oil Blend 12

BODY LOTION RECIPES 13

    Scar Diminishing Lotion Recipe 13

    Moisturizing Suntan Lotion 14

    Soothing Aloe Toner 15

    Soothing Foot Lotion Recipe 16

    2-In-1 Lotion 17

    Eczema Soother Recipe 18

HERBAL SALVE RECIPES 19

    Crack Salve 19

    Herbal Comfrey & Plantain Salve 20

Super –Relieving Salve.. 21

Eugenol & Calendula Salve 22

BALM RECIPES... 24

All-Round Healing Balm 24

Jasmine & Sandalwood Hair Balm 25

Moisturizing Lip Balm 26

Super-Hot Tiger Balm 27

Bronze Tinted Lip Balm.. 28

Honey Citrus Lip Balm Recipe 30

Healing Lip Gloss Recipe 31

SKIN CREAM RECIPES.. 32

Homemade Transdermal Detox Cream..................... 32

Rose & Ylang Ylang Luscious Body Cream 33

Rose Aloe Cream For Face 35

Cucumber Cream Recipe 36

Green Tea Face Cream.. 38

Gardener's Hand Cream Recipe................................. 39

Cuticle Jelly Recipe 40

Skin Butter Recipe 41

GEL RECIPES.. 43

Simple DIY Aloe Vera Gel... 43

Invigorating Neck Gel 44

Flax Seed & Aloe Hair Gel 45

WHIPPED BODY BUTTER RECIPES 47

Coconut Oil & Herbal Homemade Body Butter 47

Rich Whipped Body Butter 49

CLEANSERS AND MASKS 50

All-Round Lemon Cleanser 50

Skin-Revitalizing Orange Peel 51

Strawberry/Milk Facial Mask 52

Avocado Body Mask 53

INTRODUCTION

Skin care is an age-old practice that dates back to ancient Egypt. Royalties such as Cleopatra and Nefertiti are renowned for their meticulous beauty techniques and practices.

The milk bath, for instance, was Cleopatra's pastime and the result of this regular practice was a very smooth and healthy skin. Queen Nefertiti, known for her elegant beauty was fascinated with makeup, cosmetics and their natural applications almost to a point of obsession.

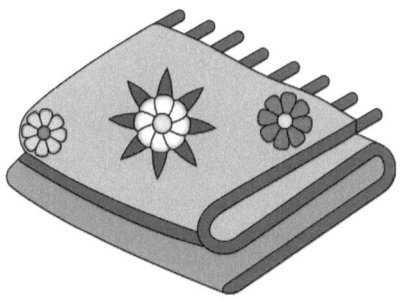

It is the same today. Everyone wants to have a healthy skin. The only difference is that majority resort to store-bought products which often contained chemicals that may be detrimental to the overall objective. According to the Environmental Working Group, the cosmetic industry has tested only 11 percent of cosmetic ingredients for safety. So what happens to the other 81%?

1

The skin is the largest and most vital eliminative organ in the body. Therefore, it ought to be attended to with utmost priority. As an important eliminative organ, it helps to detoxify about a quarter of the body's toxic substances and defend it against environmental invaders.

Our responsibility is to maintain optimal health by detoxifying daily and keeping our skin free from small openings, cracks and scratches that will pave way for harmful forces to enter into our bodies. To achieve this, we need to be mindful of the skin and body care products we regularly apply by resorting to natural products and avoiding store- bought ones as much as possible.

A number of products can be created to keep the skin soft and healthy. Creams and lotions, for instance, augment the protective barrier of the skin when it is applied. This way, the skin loses less water through evaporation, making it feel smoother and softer. We depend on these skin care products more because as we advance in age, our skin reduces the natural oil it generates.

Another reason to use homemade skin care products is their therapeutic benefits. They contain natural ingredients which benefits the body in a lot of ways. They also absorb quickly and are less expensive.

Within the confines of your kitchen, you can create your own all-natural, therapeutic skin and body products and continue the practice that started thousands of years ago.

Making Your Products Safe

Homemade beauty products are safe to the extent that we apply safe practices when making them. Here are six essential tips to ensure safety when making these products

1. Avoid Light.

Exposing your products to direct sunlight and UV rays and can cause more harm than good. Avoid exposure to light by keeping products in dark cabinets and containers.

2. Avoid Contamination.

Choose your package carefully. This way, you avoid contamination. Old containers should be sterilized and completely dried before reusing them. Never touch lip balms with your fingers. Use a cotton swab instead. Keep products bacteria from your fingers, from moisture and from heat.

3. Consider The Products' Shelf Life.

Homemade beauty products do not last as long as store-bought ones. That said, it is important to consider the shelf life of every recipe and stick to it. One way to do this is to make just what you can use in one batch and no more. Some homemade products with food in them can be refrigerated for at least a week. For non- foods products, however, the shelf-life will depend on the ingredients.

4. Use Your Sense Of Smell.

Play safe! Use your sense of smell and discard whatever smells funny or fishy.

5. Water And Homemade Beauty Products Aren't Friends.

Bacteria love to thrive in wet environments. Therefore, use clean and dry hands when applying products that involve your hand.

6. Use Natural Preservative

Extend the shelf life of your homemade products by using natural preservatives such as antioxidants and anti-microbials.

Natural Preservatives

<u>Antioxidants</u>

Antioxidants slow down the rate of oxidation. That way, oils do not go rancid but remain fresh when antioxidants are added to them. Antioxidants work really well for formulas containing fragile oils such as evening primrose, sweet or avocado. Lotions, scrubs lip balms, creams and any other product with oils in them will last longer and be more effective with the inclusion of an antioxidant.

Some natural antioxidants:

Vitamin E – contains gamma tocopherols. While Vitamin E oils are the more common one, T-50 Vitamin E Oil is larger in amounts contained.

Rosemary Oil Extract – use this natural antioxidant at a ratio rate of .15 to .5 % of the total formula.

<u>Anti-Microbials:</u>

Anti-Microbials help to destroy harmful bacteria and extend the shelf life of homemade beauty products.

Some natural anti-microbials are:

Grapefruit Seed Extract: an excellent preservative in skin care products. It should be used at a ratio of .5 – 1% ratio of the entire formula.

Coconut Oil: a very common ingredient in homemade products, it contains lauric acid, caprylic acid, antimicrobial lipids and capric acid which have antibacterial , antifungal and antiviral properties.

Essential oils provide therapeutic benefits. These benefits have been researched, confirmed and documented. However, you should do your own skin testing to ensure compliance with these ingredients.

Some of these essential oils are caraway, clove, cinnamon, tea tree, cumin, lavender, eucalyptus, lemon, rose, sage, rosemary, sandalwood and thyme. The level of result is determined by the quality and amount of the oils that are used.

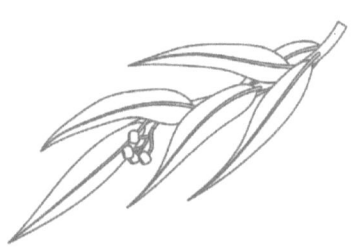

BATH RECIPES

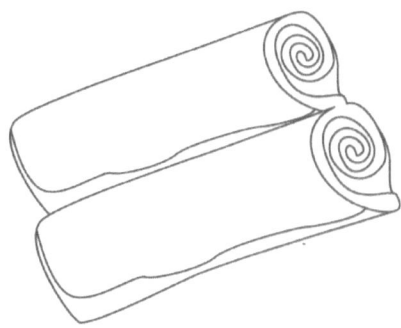

Mud Bath

Mud is rich in minerals and natural substances that are beneficial to the complexion. A well known natural beauty treatment, it is renowned for its healing powers. It tightens the skin when applied and reduces wrinkles as well.

A mud bath will provide you with a great complexion; it will rejuvenate the mind, soul and body. Also, it will detoxify the skin, ease muscle pain and tension, and reduce inflammation.

Instructions

1. Combine mud and peat with water to create a paste.

2. Slather over face and body, taking care not to get into eyes or other body orifices.

3. Let it stay for 15-30 minutes or for as long as desired.

4. Rinse off and then wrap up in warm towels.

5. Alternatively, add essential oils or Epsom salts to deepen the relaxation effects.

Baking & Sea Salt Soda Detox Baths

This bath is therapeutic for any exposure to environmental radiation, x-rays, plane flights or airport screenings by T.S.A.

<u>Instructions</u>

1. Dissolve 1pound sea salt and 1 pound baking soda to a regular sized water tub.

2. Make it as hot as you can bear.

3. Relax in the bath for about 45 minutes or until the water cools.

4. If the water is too hot to stand, add a little cold water so you can stay for at least 30 minutes.

5. Do not add more hot water however, after entering the bath.

6. Towel dry, do not shower or rinse after bath is complete.

7. Have this bath before bedtime as it is likely to make you tired.

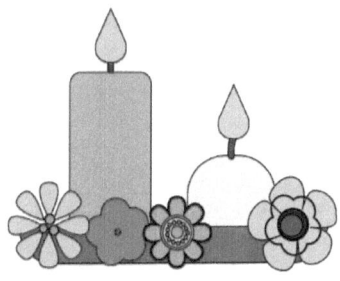

Apple Cider Vinegar (ACV) Detox Baths

This bath addresses muscle aches and pains caused by physical exertion. It is also helpful for people with Candida issues that affect the skin because it returns the skin to an optimal, slightly acidic ph. making it a difficult environment for Candida to thrive.

Furthermore, an ACV cleansing bath offers relief for individuals with arthritis, joint problems, gout, tendonitis or bursitis. It also is extremely helpful for people with excessive body odor problems

Instructions

1. Add 2 cups apple cider vinegar to a tub of water (regular size).

2. Make it as hot as you can bear.

3. Relax in the bath for about 45 minutes or until the water cools.

4. Towel dry and do not shower for 8-10 hours.

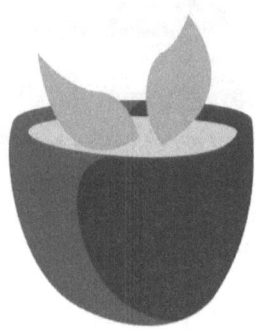

Skin Softening Milk Bath

Ingredients

3 tablespoons Epsom salt

1 cup buttermilk

3 drops lavender essential oil

½ tablespoon olive oil

Instructions

1. Combine all ingredients.

2. Pour into tub of warm water as tub fills.

3. Soak in the tub for 15-20 minutes.

4. Wash off afterwards.

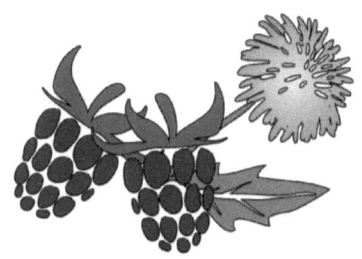

Baking Soda Detox Baths

This bath is helpful for exposure to irradiated food, sore throat, swollen glands or soreness of the mouth and gums. It also helps those with digestive impairment.

Instructions

1. Dissolve 4 cups of baking soda (aluminum free) in a regular size tubful of water.

2. Make it as hot as you can bear.

3. Relax in the bath for about 45 minutes or until the water cools.

4. Towel dry. Do not rinse after bath.

Muscle Relaxing Bath Oil Blend

<u>Ingredients</u>

2 ounces jojoba or almond oil

7 drops Rosemary

8 drops Lavender

5 drops Eucalyptus

<u>Instructions</u>

1. Combine all ingredients.

2. Pour into tub of warm water as tub fills.

3. Soak in the tub for 15 minutes.

BODY LOTION RECIPES

Scar Diminishing Lotion Recipe
Helps to lighten all kinds of scars

Ingredients

6 tsp. Jojoba Oil

7 tsp. Cocoa Butter

5 drops Frankincense Essential Oil

1 tsp. Rosehip Oil

4 drops Lavender Essential Oil

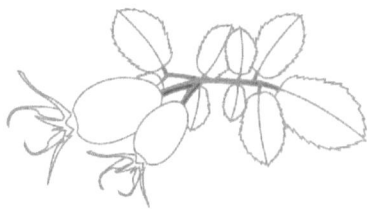

Instructions:

1. Melt the Cocoa Butter.

2. Add the rosehip and jojoba oils, mixing thoroughly.

3. Once mixture cools, mix in the essential oils.

4. Allow to it sit overnight.

5. Use on scars two times day.

Moisturizing Suntan Lotion

<u>Ingredients</u>

2 oz coconut oil

12 oz sesame oil

4.5 oz glycerin

5 capsules Vitamin E

3 oz emulsifying wax

2.5 oz cocoa butter

1 tsp citric acid

2 oz grapefruit seed extract

38 oz water (room temperature)

<u>Instructions:</u>

1. In a double boiler over medium heat, melt cocoa butter, oils and wax.

2. Add the citric acid. Take out from heat and transfer to large mixing bowl.

3. Using a stick blender, add water slowly until well blended.

4. Add vitamin E and glycerin. Cool slightly and then add GSE.

5. If desired, add fragrance. Put in containers

Soothing Aloe Toner
Soothing and refreshing light toner

<u>Ingredients</u>

1 cup aloe Vera gel

2 tbsp vitamin E oil

2 tbsp chamomile tea

5 drops peppermint essential oil

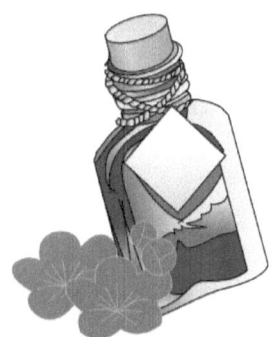

<u>Instructions:</u>

1. Combine the chamomile tea and aloe Vera gel.

2. Slowly heat in a double boiler.

3. Cool and then strain off any solids. Add the peppermint oils and vitamin E and then stir.

4. Pour into a bottle. Makes about 9 oz.

Soothing Foot Lotion Recipe

<u>Ingredients</u>

1 tbsp sweet almond

20 drops eucalyptus essential oil

10 drops tea tree essential oil

20 drops peppermint essential oil

1 cup lotion base

1 tsp Vitamin E Oil

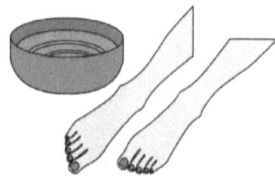

<u>Instructions:</u>

1. Mix all ingredients together.

2. Stir and put in glass container.

2-In-1 Lotion

Tanning and Moisturizing Lotion

<u>Ingredients</u>

4 oz distilled water

1 oz Shea butter

1 oz cocoa butter

1 oz organic coconut oil

2 tablespoons hemp seed oil

2 tablespoons emulsifying wax

1 teaspoon strawberry flavor oil

1 teaspoon vanilla flavor oil

2 tablespoons meadow foam oil

<u>Instructions:</u>

1. Mix the ingredients, except the flavor oils and then heat to 180 degrees or for 20- 30 minutes.

2. Blend several times during the heating cycle.

3. Cool to about 130 degrees then add the flavor oils. Stir and pour.

4. This makes about 9 oz's of tanning lotion.

Eczema Soother Recipe

A highly effective oil combination for eczema sufferers, this recipe will also keep the skin very dry and nicely lubricated.

Ingredients:

4 oz jojoba oil

20 drops evening primrose oil

12 drops roman chamomile essential oil

12 drops lavender essential oil

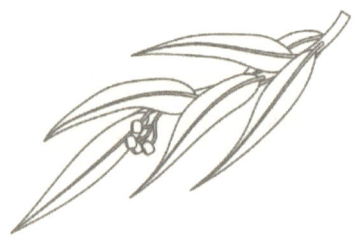

Instructions:

1. Mix all ingredients together.

2. Apply to affected areas or use as a daily skin lubricant.

3. Exceptionally good for children with eczema.

HERBAL SALVE RECIPES

Crack Salve
Treat those awful cracks on your fingernails with this salve recipe.

Ingredients

1 oz beeswax

1 oz of plantain infused olive oil

1 oz St. Johnswort infused olive oil

1 oz of calendula infused olive oil

6 drops Vitamin E

5 drops chamomile essential oil (German)

5 drops of pine needle essential oil

5 drops of tea tree essential oil

5 drops of lavender essential oil

Instructions

1. Melt together oils and beeswax

2. Once melted, add the other ingredients.

3. Let it cool and pour into clean jars.

Herbal Comfrey & Plantain Salve
For burns

Ingredients

1 oz organic comfrey leaf

1 cup organic extra virgin olive oil

1 ounce organic plantain leaf

1 ounce organic calendula flowers

1 ounce beeswax

1 ounce organic St. John's wort flowers

50 drops of lavender essential oil

Instructions

1. Pour the olive oil in top pan of a double boiler. Add the dried herbs.

2. Heat for 60 minutes over low heat.

3. Take out from heat. Next, strain and compost the herbs, setting aside the infused oil.

4. Melt the beeswax in a pan over low heat.

5. Once beeswax melts, add the lavender essential oil and herbal infused oil, mixing well.

6. Pour salve quickly in glass jars. Leave to cool before placing lids on. Label

Super –Relieving Salve *(For itches relief)*

For fresh herbs, gently spray clean and let wilt in a dry place overnight.

Ingredients

1/2 handful of chamomile heads

1 handful of chickweed

2 tbsp thyme

1/2 handful of calendula heads

2 tbsp marshmallow root

2 tbsp comfrey root

Instructions

1. Cover with olive oil and infuse over low heat for 3 hours.

2. Pass through strainer and add 1/2 oz. beeswax and1/2 oz. cocoa butter, heating until it melts.

3. Pour into containers. To test if how hard it is, drop a little on a plate. Add a little more beeswax if it is not hardened enough and then retest.

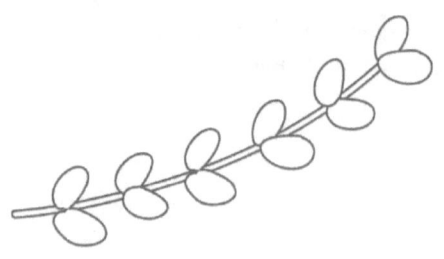

Eugenol & Calendula Salve

Lemon Balm contains Eugenol, an oily and colorless liquid which eases pain. Calendula is very soothing and works well with all types of skin conditions.

Ingredients

2 cups olive oil

3/4 cup calendula and lemon balm (equal amounts)

Instructions

1. Mix together and place in double boiler top.

2. Simmer 2 hours over low heat. (If water in bottom pot gets low, replace).

3. Pass herbs through strainer.

4. In separate pan, melt 1 tsp. lanolin or cocoa butter and 2 tsp. beeswax.

5. Add this mixture to the infused oil and stir until it cools.

6. To make this salve antibacterial, add a few drops of thyme or tea tree essential oil once it cools.

7. Put into jars. Label!

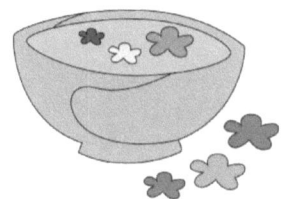

BALM RECIPES

All-Round Healing Balm
Lavender is topically healing while peppermint is cooling

Ingredients

1 part peppermint leaves

1 part lavender flowers

3 ounces of sunflower oil

2 oz coconut oil or cocoa butter

2 ounces beeswax

2 tsp peppermint & lavender essential oil

Instructions

1. Steep in lavender flowers and peppermint leaves in sunflower oil for about 45 minutes and then strain.

2. Melt coconut oil or cocoa butter in double boiler or microwave. Add the beeswax and then melt together.

3. Add the strained sunflower oil, mixing thoroughly. Once mixture cools, add the essential oil.

4. Pour into small plastic container.

Jasmine & Sandalwood Hair Balm

This moisturizing and smoothing balm will address frizz and split ends. This all-natural recipe, packed with nourishing oils will smooth your hair and cuticle, add a deep shine to it and fortify your lovely locks.

Ingredients

10 grams beeswax

10 grams Shea butter

20 grams coconut oil

10 grams sweet almond oil

1 ml rosemary extract

1 ml vitamin E oil

10 grams wheat germ oil

50 drops of aura cacia essential oil

Instructions

1. In a small glass measuring cup, combine the beeswax, Shea butter, coconut oil, wheat germ oil and sweet almond oil and place mixture in a simmering pot of water.

2. Melt over low heat. Remove and stir in the Rosemary Extract and Vitamin E Oil.

3. Add essential oil and transfer to a heat safe container. Label and apply.

Moisturizing Lip Balm

<u>Ingredients:</u>

1 1/2 tsp Shea butter

1 1/2 tsp beeswax

1/2 tsp jojoba oil

1/2 tsp sweet almond oil

3-4 drops peppermint oil or sweet orange oil

10 drops vitamin E 1000 IU

<u>Instructions:</u>

1. Melt together Shea butter, beeswax and oils in a double boiler. Take out from heat.

2. Once slightly cooled, add essential oil and vitamin E.

3. Stir and pour into containers. Let them solidify.

4. If too hard, add some sweet almond or jojoba oil. Makes about 5 tubes.

Super-Hot Tiger Balm

This recipe relieves pain by increasing the blood circulation. Camphor oils increase the blood flow on the skin surface, giving the balm its hot feeling and reducing pain to provide relief. This balm soothes ailments like respiratory problems, headaches muscle, neck and joint pain and arthritis.

Ingredients:

4g peppermint essential oil

2g cassia essential oil

5g menthol essential oil

5g camphor essential oil

26g cocoa butter

6g cajeput essential oil

4g chili seed essential oil

26g beeswax

Instructions:

1. Combine all the essential oils in a container. Warm the essential oils gently by placing container in a very hot water bath.

2. In a small saucepan, combine beeswax and cocoa butter and melt over medium low heat.

3. Once melted, remove essential oils from hot water bath and dry container.

4. Pour beeswax mixture straight into the essential oils, stirring to mix well.

5. Decant the melted mixture quickly into smaller glass jars or leave to cool in Mason jars.

Bronze Tinted Lip Balm

A shimmery moisturizing lip balm with a sheer bronze tint color!

Ingredients:

2 tsp beeswax

2 1/2 tsp coconut oil

1 tsp mango butter

1/2 tsp cocoa butter

1/2 tsp vitamin E oil

1 tsp sweet almond oil

1/2 tsp castor oil

1 tsp kukui nut oil

1/4 tsp amber mica

1 tsp aloe Vera oil

Flavor oil (optional)

Instructions:

1. In a double boiler, mix together all oils and butter and melt over gentle heat.

2. Once melted, remove from heat. Add flavor oil and then add the amber mica, stirring to blend thoroughly.

3. Pour into tubes. Allow to cool and set.

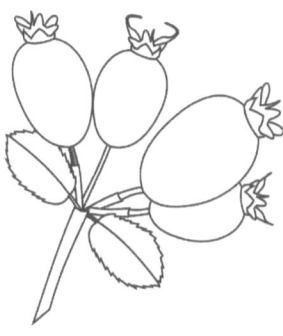

Honey Citrus Lip Balm Recipe

Honey acts as an astringent. It tightens the pores, reduces wrinkles and is also good for acne.

Ingredients:

1/4 cup almond oil

1/8 tsp. glycerin (vegetable)

1/8 tsp vitamin E 250 IU or higher

1 tsp honey

1/2 oz. beeswax

5 drops grapefruit essential oil

5 drops lemon essential oil

5 drops orange essential oil

Instructions:

1. Warm almond oil, glycerin, beeswax and vitamin E in a small saucepan until the beeswax melts.

2. Add essential oils and stir.

3. Finally, pour into lip balm containers.

4. The essential oils are phototoxic so do not apply before going out into the sun.

Healing Lip Gloss Recipe

Heals chapped lips & keeps it glossy.

<u>Ingredients:</u>

1/2 tsp jojoba oil

1/4 tsp meadowfoam oil

1/2 tsp coconut oil

1 tsp castor oil

1 tsp beeswax

1/2 tsp cocoa butter

2-3 drops peppermint essential oil

<u>Instructions:</u>

1. Melt together all oils in a double boiler (less peppermint).

2. Stir in peppermint essential oil and pour into containers. Leave to cool.

SKIN CREAM RECIPES

Homemade Transdermal Detox Cream

Zeolite, the most powerful detox agent is a primary ingredient of any transdermal detox cream. In the body, it attracts toxins such as, chemicals, radiation, free radicals and heavy metals into its structure and excretes them via natural bodily functions.

As a result, the body gradually becomes less toxic, leading to healthier natural repair functions and immune system improvement.

Ingredients:

1 cup micronized zeolite (4ppm or smaller)

1 cup Cacao butter (raw, organic, fair-trade)

1 cup extra virgin coconut oil (cold-pressed, raw & organic)

Instructions:

1. Melt coconut oil and cacao butter at low heat using a bain-marie.

2. Add the zeolite

3. Lastly, pour in a jar and seal

Rose & Ylang Ylang Luscious Body Cream

<u>Ingredients:</u>

Oil Phase:

1 1/2 tablespoon infused alkanet oil

1/2 tbsp + 1 tsp Shea butter

1/2 tbsp + 1 tsp macadamia nut oil

1/2 tbsp + 1/4 tsp virgin coconut oil

1/2 tsp stearic acid

1 1/2 tbsp vegetable emulsifying wax

5 drops rosemary oil extract

10 drops vitamin E oil

 Water Phase:

1/2 teaspoon potassium sorbate

4 oz. rose or lavender hydrosol or distilled water

20 drops ylang-ylang essential oil

30 drops rose essential oil or attar

<u>Instructions:</u>

1. Use the double boiler method to melt the water and oil phase in two separate Pyrex measuring cups. Do this until the oils and fats are fully melted.

2. Add the water phase gently to the oil phase, beating continuously with an egg beater.

3. Once the mixture starts to thicken, add red colorant until a nice shade of pink is achieved

3. Lastly, add the essential oils, gently beating in. Pour into containers and leave to thicken.

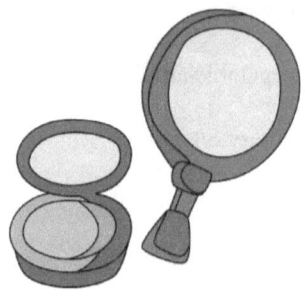

Rose Aloe Cream For Face

<u>Ingredients:</u>

3 tbsp of rice bran oil

1 ½ tsp of extra virgin coconut oil

1 3/4 tsp jasmine or orange water

1/4 tsp lanolin

1 3/4 tsp illipe butter

1/2 tsp beeswax

3/4/ tsp vegetable glycerin

2 tbsp of rose hydrosol

1 tbsp aloe Vera gel

1 vitamin A capsule

1 vitamin E capsule

<u>Instructions:</u>

1. Melt the lanolin, beeswax, butter and oils mixture over medium heat.

2. Let mixture cool to room temperature. (To have a successful cream, the water and oil mixtures must be of equal temperature).

3. Put the floral water and hydrosol, vitamin E and A, glycerin and aloe Vera into a blender.

4. Turn the speed on medium-high then gradually drizzle in the oil mixture. Keep at it until all the oil is added. (The mixture should look creamy and thick).

5. Refrigerate cream. Cream will stay 2-3 weeks of kept in the bathroom. However, adding a preservative will extend the shelf-life.

Cucumber Cream Recipe

Cucumber helps to smoothes, nourish and cleanse the skin. They also help to reduce wrinkles and fine lines, leaving a glowing complexion. Cucumber juice supports the liver in cleansing.

Ingredients:

1 tbsp fresh cucumber juice

¼ tsp borax powder

¼ cup fractionated coconut oil

1 tbsp beeswax

1 tbsp distilled water

8 drops grapefruit seed extract

Emerald mica or jade for color (optional)

Cucumber fragrance oil (optional)

Instructions:

1. Dissolve the borax in the distilled water. To it, add the grapefruit seed extract.

2. In another cup, mix oil and beeswax together. Place the cup in a pan of about 1-2 inches of water

3. Heat the oil-beeswax mixture over medium heat in the water bath until beeswax is melted, stir occasionally. Bring mixture almost to boiling.

4. Remove mixture from water bath. Add the borax-water mixture gently to it. Add the cucumber juice, stirring well.

5. Add fragrance oil if using and leave to cool.

6. Take a small quantity of cream, mix the mica into it well to remove all the clumps.

7. Add the now colored cream to the main batch, blending well.

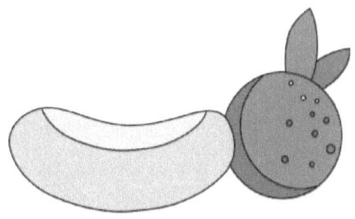

Green Tea Face Cream

Green tea works by helping to repair sun damage and reduce aging signs. The Rose hip seed oil deals with skin regeneration and repair and regeneration. Almond and Coconut oils are excellent moisturizers. In short, this recipe smells delicious and does wonders to your skin!

<u>Ingredients:</u>

1 packet organic green tea

.25 oz beeswax (grated, or in pellets)

1 oz almond oil

1/4 tsp Rose Hip Seed Oil

1 oz coconut oil

<u>Instructions:</u>

1. In a double boiler, combine oils and wax and oils and melt.

2. Open the tea bag. Pour loose tea directly into the oils. Allow mixture to get warm and extract from tea for 15 minutes.

3. Using a fine mesh sieve, strain the oil mixture into a deep cup (Pyrex measuring cup).

4. Whip mixture with a hand mixer, scraping down the sides occasionally, until creamy and room temperature.

5. Store cream in a cool dark place.

Gardener's Hand Cream Recipe
Added protection for working in the garden

<u>Ingredients:</u>

2 tbs. avocado oil

2 tsp. glycerin

1 tbs. honey

1 1/2 cups finely ground almonds

<u>Instructions:</u>

1. In a ceramic bowl, mix the avocado oil, glycerin and honey thoroughly.

2. Add an adequate amount of almonds to form a paste.

3. To apply to hands, rub in very well until it penetrates the skin and the almond remains fall off.

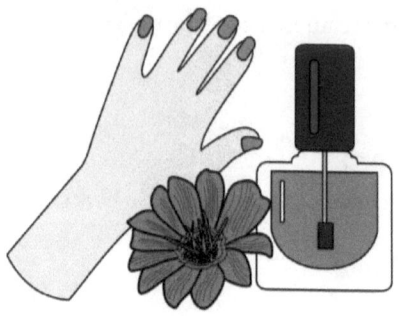

Cuticle Jelly Recipe

A softening jelly for your cuticles

<u>Ingredients:</u>

2 grams beeswax

30 grams grape seed oil

5 grams avocado oil

5 grams sweet almond butter

8 grams evening primrose oil

30 grams sunflower oil

5 grams hemp oil

8 grams lanolin

8 grams walnut oil

5 grams Illipe butter

1 gram fragrance oil

1 gram Vitamin E oil

Instructions:

1. Combine ingredients and melt. Do not overheat.

2. Once melted, add the vitamin E oil and any desired essential oils.

3. Fill bottles.

Skin Butter Recipe
Thick moisturizer for dry skin

Ingredients:

1 oz olive or coconut oil

2 oz Shea butter

1/2 oz meadowfoam

1/2 oz jojoba oil

2-3 drops essential of choice

Instructions:

1. Mix all ingredients together thoroughly.

2. To revitalize cracked &dry skin on heels of feet, apply at night and cover feet in socks.

3. Skin will be soft and smooth in the morning.

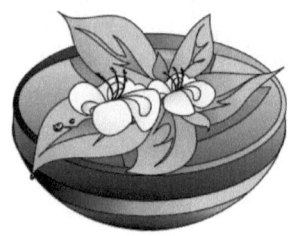

GEL RECIPES

Simple DIY Aloe Vera Gel

This gel contains anti-fungal, antibacterial and antiviral properties. A powerful anti aging moisturizer, it heals sunburn, insect bites, acne, eczema and stretch marks.

<u>Ingredients</u>

¼ cup aloe Vera pulp (six leaves of 4 to 6 ")

1 tbsp coconut oil

4 drops lemon grass essential oil

6 drops tea tree oil

<u>Instructions</u>

1. Cut leaves from plant. Put them in a bowl at an upright standing of 45 degree angle. Leave for 1 hour.

2. Wash the leaves. Cut off thorns on both sides and peel 1 side (use a potato peeler). Scrape off the gel from leaves with a knife.

3. Blend gel in a blender until slightly fluffy. Add remaining ingredients and blend well. Pour into a clean container.

4. Last for 3 months

Invigorating Neck Gel

Ingredients:

15 drops Peppermint Essential Oil

2 oz Aloe Vera Gel (unscented)

Instructions:

1. Mix the aloe Vera gel and oil in a small jar until it becomes cloudy.

2. Apply a small amount to the back of your neck and massage.

3. This recipe will provide relief to your neck giving it a cooling sensation that will last for some minutes.

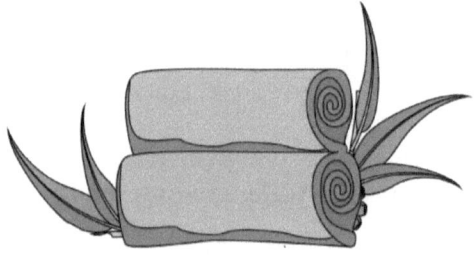

Flax Seed & Aloe Hair Gel

Give your hair volume and help to hold it in a natural shape with this recipe.

Ingredients:

1 tbsp Flax Seed

2 tbsp Aloe Vera

5 drops of Ylang Ylang Essential Oils

1 cup of Water

Instructions:

1. Fit a knee-high nylon over the edge of a pint sized Mason jar. (Let most of nylon foot be inside the jar). Set it to the side of a stove top. You will be using this to strain the flax seeds from your hair gel.

2. Bring the water to boil in a saucepan for 1 minute and lower heat.

3. Add the flax seed and keep boiling for 3- 5 minutes, until the mixture becomes thick and attains an egg white consistency.

4. Turn off the heat, stir in the Aloe Vera and pour the mixture into the nylon that is inside of the Mason jar.

5. Tightly twist the nylon from the top down, being careful as the mixture is hot. (You can tie a knot in the nylon top so the flax seed doesn't keep coming back out the open top).

6. Squeeze the mixture out of the nylon with tongs into the Mason jar.

7. Add the essential oil. Let mixture cool then transfer to a dispensing bottle

8. To use, massage 1-2 tsp into damp hair and style as usual.

9. This yields approximately 8 ounces hair gel.

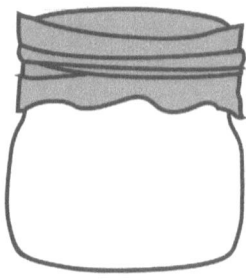

WHIPPED BODY BUTTER RECIPES

Coconut Oil & Herbal Homemade Body Butter
Valuable in the cold winter time when the skin gets really dry

Ingredients:

2 tbsp solid Shea butter

1 tbsp mint infused coconut oil

1 tbsp olive oil

1 ml vitamin E (or 1 capsule)

Dried rose petals, fresh rosemary

7 drops each lavender essential oil& lime essential oil

Instructions:

1. In a double boiler, melt Shea butter and coconut oil.

2. Add the vegetable oil and some dried or fresh herbs, if desired

3. If using herbs, heat mixture for 20 minutes, then carefully strain and squeeze out oil completely from the herbs. If not, proceed to the next step once the butters melt.

4. Remove from heat, cool. Add the vitamin E and essential oils.

5. Whip butter until thick and fluffy for 5-10 minutes.

6. Transfer body butter to jars with the help of a spatula.

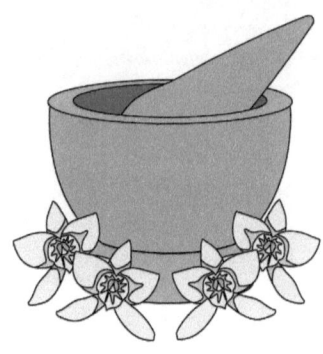

Rich Whipped Body Butter

Let your skin drink up the nutrient-dense goodness from these oils

Ingredients

1 cup of cocoa butter

1/2 cup coconut oil

1/2 cup of jojoba oil

Instructions:

1. Use a double boiler to melt coconut oil and cocoa butter gently until totally liquid.

2. Add the jojoba. Refrigerate for several hours until the oil mixture starts to firm, but hasn't turned completely solid.

3. Whip the semi-solid mixture with a hand mixer until white peaks form.

4. Scoop into glass jars. Chill for 1 hour in the fridge.

CLEANSERS AND MASKS

All-Round Lemon Cleanser

Lemons are a natural source of antioxidants and alpha hydroxyl acids (AHAs) which tones, cleanses and exfoliates the skin.

Ingredients

1 tsp lemon juice

2 tbsp milk or cream

1/8 cup ground almonds

Instructions:

1. Combine thoroughly. Gently cleanse skin.

2. Rinse with warm water.

Skin-Revitalizing Orange Peel

Oranges are a great source of vitamin C and AHAs, which are clinically proven to prevent fine lines and wrinkles. The egg yolk and honey moisturizes and the citrus juice exfoliates the dead skin cells, stimulating new cell production.

Ingredients

1/8 cup fresh citrus (orange, lemon or lime) juice

1 egg yolk

1 packet plain gelatin

1 tsp honey

Instructions:

1. Combine thoroughly. Apply to skin.

2. Leave for 20 to 25 minutes. Wash off

Strawberry/Milk Facial Mask

The natural antioxidants in strawberries help to repair skin and protect it from environmental stress. Additionally, the salicylic acid in strawberries eliminates dead skin cells, revealing a smooth and radiant skin.

Ingredients

1/2 cup fresh strawberries

1 tablespoon fresh milk

1 tablespoon rice flour or cornstarch

Instructions:

1. Mash together all ingredients to make a smooth paste.

2. Spread over your face and neck, and leave on for 20 minutes.

3. Rinse with warm water and pat your skin dry. Use twice weekly.

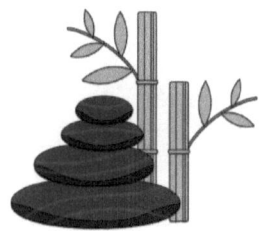

Avocado Body Mask

Avocados have anti-aging properties. It contains vitamins A, D and E, proteins, lecithin and beta-carotene which helps to fight cancer. They work to reduce age spots, scars and heal sun-damaged skin.

Ingredients

2 avocados, thoroughly mashed into a paste

3 tablespoons sea salt or kosher salt

1/4 cup honey

Grated rind of 2 fresh lemons (juice inclusive)

1/4 cup organic coconut oil

Instructions:

1. Mix all until smooth and creamy.

2. Apply to skin for 10 -15 minutes,

3. Scrub off with warm water.

4. Refrigerate unused portions for 2-3 days.